THE NURSE
I AM BECOMING

The Nurse
I Am Becoming

A Guided Reflection Companion for Nursing Students
Developing Clinical Judgment, Confidence,
and Professional Identity

Nancy S. Ferrell Jones, DNP, RN

ISBN: 979-8-9953386-0-4

Printed in the United States of America

This Journal Belongs To

Name

Semester

Year

TABLE OF CONTENTS

TABLE OF CONTENTS
(continued)

Professional Identity — Weeks 21–34

Closing

Professional Guidance

DEDICATION

This book is dedicated first to my nursing students —
especially my first cohort —
who trusted me with their questions, their fears, and their becoming.

You reminded me why standing in the gap matters.
You know who you are.

To my husband and sons — my anchor, joy, and my reason.

To my mother and brother — my light.

To my granddaddy, whose life of service shaped my wisdom and
legacy.

To my band director, who taught me excellence and command.

To those who quietly supported my family and me —
your presence mattered more than you know.

IN MEMORIAM

To my grandmother, Momma —
a woman of elegance, discipline, and innovation.
A graduate of Madam C. J. Walker's College of Beauty Culture,
a business leader who modeled poise, excellence, and command.

Her legacy of entrepreneurship, stewardship, and dignity lives on in
me.

To my father —
a brilliant mind, a man of discipline and service,
whose strength and leadership set a standard long before I understood
it.

To my grandfather —
a trailblazer who served as both police officer and jailer,
whose courage and leadership paved the way for generations beyond
his own.

AUTHOR'S NOTE

When my first cohort of nursing students began their journey, they arrived determined. Energetic. Ready to learn. Hopeful. Like every student entering a demanding professional program, they carried both excitement and uncertainty — and they showed up anyway.

I am a Black woman in nursing. I know what it means to navigate spaces where your presence is rare and your voice is sometimes overlooked. I was a Certified Nursing Aide for ten years while pursuing my nursing degree and my first degree in psychology. I never gave up on becoming a nurse — and the journey taught me more than any classroom ever could.

The statistics are stark. Black nurses represent a small percentage of the overall nursing workforce. Those in leadership positions — directors, executives, advanced practice leaders — represent an even smaller fraction. Black nurses with a Doctor of Nursing Practice degree in executive leadership make up approximately two percent of the field. When I was a nursing student, the number of Black students in my cohort was already limited. As an educator, I watched that number grow even smaller.

Representation matters — not just in the classroom, but in mentorship, in leadership, and in the spaces where decisions are made about who belongs in this profession. When a student sees someone who looks like them, who understands their culture, their burden, and their experience, something shifts. They begin to believe they belong. That belief is not a luxury. It is a clinical necessity.

During my time teaching, I observed something important: nursing education demands everything from students. You learn complex science, develop clinical judgment, and grow into the professional and emotional responsibilities that come with caring for others. And you do all of this while navigating your own life — your family, your finances, your fears, your doubts, and your quiet determination to keep going.

Some learning environments support that journey. Others make it harder.

This guided reflection companion was created for every student who has ever questioned whether they could continue. For those who have felt unseen in a classroom. For those carrying the weight of representation. For the student balancing a family, a job, and a full course load. For the CNA who has been working bedside for years and finally made it into a nursing program.

For the phlebotomist, the medical technician, the EMT — everyone in the healthcare pipeline who is moving toward nursing and needs to know that someone prepared this space for them.

I also wrote this for the student who has encountered an environment that was not built to hold them. Who has sat in a classroom and felt afraid to ask a question. Who has navigated the emotional weight of a difficult learning experience while still showing up every single day and doing the work. You are not alone. What you experienced has happened before — and there is a way through it.

This experience is for them. And for every student who comes after.

Whether you are in your first semester or your last, beginning a new clinical rotation or preparing for licensure, working as a healthcare professional and dreaming of nursing school, or a practicing nurse continuing to evolve — this companion is yours. It is a tool. It is a companion. It is a reminder that someone, somewhere, understood what you would face before you ever opened this page.

You are becoming. That journey deserves to be witnessed and honored.

This guided experience will help you do both.

— Nancy S. Ferrell Jones, DNP, RN

Context Matters

Nursing school is not only an academic journey — it is an emotional and professional transition. That shift can feel both inspiring and overwhelming at the same time.

For many who enter nursing programs, this journey began long before the first day of class. Some have worked as nursing aides, phlebotomists, medical technicians, or emergency responders. They have already stood beside patients. They have already learned to care. And yet nursing school asks them to begin again — to unlearn some habits, to build new ones, and to grow into a clinical identity that is still forming. That process is not a step backward. It is a deepening.

In the early weeks of a nursing program, students often experience a mixture of excitement, pressure, and uncertainty. They are learning new language, new expectations, and new responsibilities while trying to build confidence in unfamiliar environments.

As the semester progresses, the emotional rhythm of the experience becomes more complex. Clinical days bring moments of pride and learning, but they can also bring self-doubt, comparison with peers, and the quiet pressure to perform well.

For many students, these experiences happen while they are also balancing families, jobs, financial pressures, and personal responsibilities. Very few people outside of nursing education fully understand the weight students carry during this time.

Recognizing this context matters because growth rarely happens in perfect conditions. It happens while students are navigating uncertainty, developing professional judgment, and learning how to care for others while still balancing how to care for themselves.

This companion is meant to sit beside that experience — not as another assignment, but as a grounding place to pause, think, and reconnect with the purpose that brought you into nursing.

Why This Journal Exists

This guided reflection companion was created to give nursing students something that is often missing during the intensity of nursing school: a structured space to think, process, and grow.

In most programs, students move quickly from lecture to skills labs to clinical rotations. They complete care plans, prepare for exams, and learn new procedures at a rapid pace. While these academic expectations are necessary, students are rarely given time to pause and reflect on what they are becoming through the process.

The purpose of this experience is to create that pause.

Each week offers a rhythm of affirmation, reflection, and space for personal insight. These moments are designed to help students recognize patterns in their experiences, build confidence in their developing judgment, and strengthen the professional identity that is forming throughout the semester.

This is not a guided experience about perfection or performance. It is a companion for the journey of becoming — a place where you can remember why you chose the path of nursing in the first place.

Over time, these reflections become more than notes on a page. They become a record of resilience, learning, and transformation — the quiet evidence of the nurse you are becoming.

Note to the Reader

Nursing school will stretch you in ways you may not expect. There will be moments when the pace feels relentless, when the weight of responsibility begins to settle in, and when you question whether you are truly ready for what lies ahead.

These moments are not signs that you are failing. They are often the very moments when growth begins. This companion was created to give you a place to pause in the middle of the demands of nursing education.

Each page invites you to think about the nurse you are becoming — not only through clinical skill and knowledge, but through courage, compassion, and professional identity. You do not need to fill every line perfectly. You do not need to have every answer today. What matters most is that you continue showing up.

One lesson at a time.
One skill at a time.
One moment at a time.

This professional tool is simply a companion along the way.

This experience was written for the nursing student. But if you are a CNA, a phlebotomist, a medical technician, or any healthcare professional moving toward nursing — these pages are for you too. You are already becoming. This experience simply gives that becoming a place to land.

How to Use This Journal

This guided reflection companion moves in rhythm with the real demands of nursing school.

Each week supports the work you are already doing — skills check-offs, lab practice, simulation, clinical rotations, care plans, and exams.

Use it:

• Before lecture to focus your attention
• After lab to evaluate skill development
• After clinical rotations to reflect on growth and emotional responses (no patient identifiers)
• While preparing care plans to strengthen clinical reasoning

This is not extra work.
It is structured reflection.

Nursing school moves quickly. These pages slow the pace — allowing you to think clearly, track your development, and recognize your growth.

Return to it beyond this semester — during transition, challenge, or leadership. What you record here becomes part of your professional story.

You do not have to start at Week One. If you are mid-semester, begin where you are. If you are starting a new clinical rotation, return to the early weeks — because every new clinical height is its own beginning. If you are a practicing nurse using this framework for professional development, let the language speak to wherever you are in your journey. This experience does not expire. It grows with you.

The Rhythm of This Journal

Each week in nursing school carries its own weight.

Some weeks feel steady.
Others feel heavy.
Some pass quickly.
Others linger longer than expected.

Growth does not move in straight lines.

At the beginning of each week, pause.
Notice where you are — mentally, emotionally, academically.

At the end of each week, reflect.

What strengthened you?
What challenged you?
What are you still learning to hold?

You do not need to document everything. Some weeks will require more space.

Some will only need a few purposeful lines.

There is no expectation of perfection here.

What matters is returning — again and again — to yourself within the work.

This framework is not designed to measure you. It is designed to support you.

The Nurse's Shield

The Nurse's Shield is a structured framework designed to support your development as a nurse. It represents how you think, what grounds you, what protects you, and who you are becoming in practice.

Nursing school will challenge you intellectually, emotionally, and professionally. This shield helps you organize your internal foundation so you can respond—not react—under pressure.

This is not about perfection. It is about clarity, awareness, and growth.

Each section of the shield has a specific purpose. When completed, it becomes a personal reference you can return to throughout your training and into your practice.

How to Use the Shield

Follow each section of the shield intentionally. Do not rush this process. Each area reflects a different part of your development.

TOP
Beliefs / Mindset

LEFT
Support System

CENTER
Professional Identity

RIGHT
Strengths

FOUNDATION
Values / Why

BORDER
Boundaries / Protection

Section Guidance:
- Top: What do you believe about yourself as you learn and grow?
- Left: Who supports you? (people, mentors, resources)
- Right: What strengths do you bring into nursing?
- Center: Who are you becoming as a nurse?
- Foundation: What values ground you?
- Border: What protects your peace, boundaries, and well-being?

A Note to the Student

This shield belongs to you.

What you write here does not have to last forever.
It simply reflects where you are as you begin.

Return to this page when you need clarity, when you need grounding,
or when you need to remember why you chose this path.

You are building something with care and intention.

And you do not have to build it alone.

This guided reflection companion is not about perfection.

It is about becoming.

Opening Formation Statement

This companion was written for the nursing student who walks into the classroom hopeful, determined, and quietly uncertain. Nursing school is rigorous by design. The content is demanding. The expectations are high. The responsibility is real.

But beneath the lectures, labs, clinical rotations, and exams, something deeper is taking shape.

Character.
Discipline.
Composure.
Integrity.

This framework is not simply a place to record what you learn. It is a space to witness who you are becoming while you learn it.

Each week follows the natural rise of nursing education — from foundational understanding to complex reasoning, advocacy, accountability, and leadership.

You may feel nervous. You may feel stretched. At times you may question yourself. These experiences do not disqualify you. They are part of professional formation.

Read slowly. Reflect honestly. Write openly.

Leave space for growth.

This is where formation begins.

WEEK ONE

Every Beginning Feels Like This

There is a feeling that lives in the body at the start of something important. You may know it well by now — the mixture of hope and uncertainty that arrives before a new chapter begins. The excitement that sits just beside the fear. The quiet question underneath everything: Am I ready for this?

That feeling does not belong only to first-semester nursing students. It belongs to every nurse, at every level, standing at the threshold of something new. The CNA beginning their first shift. The nursing student walking into their first clinical. The experienced RN starting a new specialty. The nurse practitioner seeing their first patient independently. The doctoral student beginning their residency.

Every beginning feels like this. The nervousness is not a sign that you are unprepared. It is a sign that what you are stepping into matters to you. And that matters.

This week — whatever week this is for you, whatever level you are entering — the most important thing is not that you feel ready. It is that you showed up. Courage is not the absence of uncertainty. It is the decision to begin anyway.

You began. That is everything.

The space below each affirmation and reflection is yours. Write freely. There are no wrong answers.

Affirmation

Every Beginning Feels Like This

I show up even when I am uncertain. Every expert was once
exactly where I am standing. I am not behind — I am beginning.
And beginning, again and again, is what becoming looks like.

Pause & Consider

Every Beginning Feels Like This

Take a few honest minutes with these questions. There are no wrong answers. Write what is true for you right now.
• What emotions did you bring into this new beginning? Name all of them honestly — the hopeful ones and the fearful ones.
• What does readiness feel like for you? Is it a feeling — or is it a decision?
• What brought you to this moment? What is the deeper reason you are here?
• What would you tell yourself right now if you were speaking from the nurse you are becoming rather than the student you feel like today?

WEEK TWO

Discipline Before Confidence

Confidence does not arrive before the work. It arrives because of it.

In the early weeks of any new nursing season, confidence may feel distant. You are learning new language, new expectations, new ways of thinking. You are building habits before you can see the results of those habits. You are preparing before you feel prepared.

This is where discipline does its quiet, important work. Discipline is not motivation. Motivation comes and goes — it is unreliable, emotional, and tied to how you feel on a given day. Discipline is different. Discipline shows up regardless of how you feel. It prepares before the exam even when the exam feels far away. It practices the skill even when the skill feels awkward. It asks the question even when asking feels vulnerable.

Every nurse who now moves through a clinical environment with ease and certainty got there by doing the small things consistently, before confidence arrived. Not after. Before.
You are building that foundation right now. Trust the process even when you cannot yet see the product.

Affirmation

Discipline Before Confidence

I do not wait for confidence before I prepare. I prepare, and confidence follows. My consistency today is building the nurse I am becoming tomorrow.

Pause & Consider

Discipline Before Confidence

- Where did you show discipline this week even when motivation was low?
- What preparation habit is beginning to work for you? What needs adjustment?
- What does it feel like in your body when you are prepared versus unprepared? How can that awareness serve you?
- Who or what is helping you stay consistent right now?

WEEK THREE

The Courage to Ask

There is a kind of courage that does not announce itself loudly. It shows up in small, important moments — like raising your hand when you do not understand something. Like sending an email to ask for clarification. Like saying, out loud, in a room full of people: I have a question.

In nursing, asking questions is not a sign of weakness. It is a clinical safety skill. The nurse who asks is the nurse who catches the error. The nurse who speaks up is the nurse who protects the patient. Learning to ask begins here — in the classroom, before it matters in the way it will one day matter at the bedside.

This week, you may have your first skills check-offs approaching. The pressure to perform correctly is real. And in that pressure, it can feel easier to stay quiet than to admit uncertainty.

Do not stay quiet. Ask. Clarify. Verify. You are building the habit that will one day save a life.

Affirmation

The Courage to Ask

Asking questions is not weakness — it is wisdom. I advocate for my learning the same way I will one day advocate for my patients. My voice belongs in every room I enter.

Pause & Consider

The Courage to Ask

• Was there a moment recently when you wanted to ask a question but held back? What stopped you?
• What would it mean for your patients one day if you learned to ask without hesitation?
• Who in your current learning environment feels safe to approach with questions? How can you lean into that relationship?
• How does asking for help reflect professional strength rather than weakness?

When You Are Being Tested

Every nursing journey has its tests. Not just the formal ones — the exams, the evaluations, the check-offs — but the internal ones too. The moments where you are asked to demonstrate what you know under pressure, in front of others, with something real at stake.

Tests arrive at every level. The student faces their first exam. The new graduate faces their first solo shift. The nurse practitioner faces their first complex case. The doctoral student faces their committee. The form changes. The feeling does not.

Here is what I want you to know before you walk into whatever test is in front of you right now: the test does not create your knowledge. It simply asks you to show what is already there. Everything you have prepared, practiced, and internalized — it belongs to you. No exam can take it away.

Tests in nursing measure more than content knowledge. They measure your ability to think clearly under pressure, to prioritize when everything feels urgent, to trust your preparation when anxiety tells you not to. Those are clinical skills. You are practicing them right now.

Walk in prepared. Walk in grounded. Whatever the result — you learn from it and you continue. That is what nurses do.

Affirmation

When You Are Being Tested

I have prepared well. I trust the knowledge I have built. I approach this test with a clear mind and a steady presence. Whatever the outcome, I learn from it and continue forward.

Pause & Consider

When You Are Being Tested

- What preparation strategies have served you best leading into this evaluation?
- How did you manage the anxiety or pressure that came with being tested? What helped?
- After the evaluation — regardless of the result — what did you learn about how you think under pressure?
- What will you do the same or differently next time?

WEEK FIVE

When Responsibility Becomes Real

There comes a point in every nursing journey when the weight of responsibility becomes undeniably real.

It is not a dramatic moment, usually. It happens quietly — in the middle of a skill, a procedure, a decision, a calculation. And something shifts. You understand, in a way that is deeper than academic, that what you are doing has consequences. That precision matters. That attention to detail is not a personality preference — it is a patient safety imperative.

This moment arrives at every level of nursing. It arrives for the student learning to administer medication for the first time. It arrives for the nurse learning a new and more complex intervention. It arrives for the advanced practice provider writing their first prescription for a controlled substance. It arrives for the nurse leader realizing that their decisions affect not one patient but hundreds.

The intensity deepens with each level. But the core truth remains the same: in nursing, what you do matters. How carefully you do it matters. The habits you build now — the precision, the verification, the willingness to slow down when speed feels expected — will protect patients you have not yet met.

Let the weight land. Do not run from it. It is what makes you a nurse.

Affirmation

When Responsibility Becomes Real

I practice precision because lives depend on it. I slow down when it
matters most. I am building habits now that will protect patients I
have not yet met. Accuracy is my act of care.

Pause & Consider

When Responsibility Becomes Real

• Where did the weight of responsibility feel most real to you this week?
• How did it feel when you understood — deeply, not just intellectually — that what you are learning has real consequences?
• What habit are you building right now that will protect your future patients?
• How does slowing down — even under pressure — reflect professional integrity?

WEEK SIX

What You Are Carrying

Nursing education was not designed with the assumption that students arrive carrying full lives.

But you do. Whatever level you are at — whatever season of nursing you are in — you are carrying more than your clinical bag. You are carrying families. Financial pressure. Relationships that require tending. Health concerns of your own or of people you love. Dreams that feel both close and impossibly far away. The weight of being the first, or the only, or the one everyone is counting on.

You carry all of this into every classroom, every clinical shift, every simulation, every exam. And very few people around you fully see it.

I want to name it clearly: the fact that you are still here — still showing up, still learning, still choosing this path — while carrying everything you are carrying, is not ordinary. It is extraordinary. It deserves to be acknowledged, not just pushed through.

The nurse who learns to carry their own weight with grace is the nurse who can hold space for patients carrying theirs. You are practicing that right now. Even in the hardest weeks. Maybe especially then.

You do not have to carry it perfectly. You just have to keep going.

Affirmation

What You Are Carrying

I acknowledge the full weight of what I am carrying. I am not weak
for finding this hard — I am strong for continuing anyway. My
endurance is building something real in me.

Pause & Consider

What You Are Carrying

• What are you carrying this week that has nothing to do with nursing school but affects everything about how you show up?
• What is one thing you can release this week, even temporarily, to protect your energy?
• Who in your life truly understands what you are going through? How can you lean on that support?
• How does learning to carry your own weight with grace prepare you to hold space for patients carrying theirs?

MIDTERM PAUSE

You are no longer at the beginning.

The pace is familiar now. The expectations are clearer. The pressure feels different than it did in the first weeks.

Before moving forward, pause here.

Notice what has settled.
Notice what has sharpened.
Notice what feels different inside you.

Midpoint is not about evaluation.
It is about awareness.

You have more information now than you did at the start.

Let that matter.

Midpoint Reflection

An Honest Inventory

You have completed exams. You have practiced skills. You have entered clinical space. You have experienced instruction from different personalities and approaches.

This is a moment for clarity.

Consider:

- What preparation habits are strengthening me?
- Where have I become more disciplined?
- How do I respond under pressure?
- What patterns are helping me succeed?
- What needs refinement moving forward?

Growth is not accidental.
It becomes visible when I look at it directly.

Midpoint is not a verdict.
It is a recalibration.

What I adjust now strengthens the remainder of this journey.

Midterm Affirmation

I recognize that I am no longer at the beginning.

I see more clearly how I prepare, how I respond, and how I carry responsibility.

I take ownership of what strengthens me and I refine what does not.

I move forward with greater awareness, greater discipline, and greater intention.

What I build from this point forward will reflect what I have learned so far.

WEEK SEVEN

When Doubt Gets Loud

Somewhere in the middle of every nursing journey, doubt gets loud.

It does not always announce itself clearly. Sometimes it sounds like fatigue. Sometimes it sounds like comparison — looking at someone else and wondering why they seem more confident, more capable, more certain than you feel. Sometimes it sounds like a quiet voice that says: maybe this is not for me.

Hear this clearly: doubt is not evidence. It is a feeling. And feelings, even powerful and persistent ones, are not facts.

Doubt visits every nurse, at every level. It visits the student who passed their last exam but cannot remember why they know anything. It visits the experienced RN starting a new specialty and feeling like a beginner again. It visits the nurse practitioner in their first year of independent practice. It visits the doctoral student wondering if they belong in academic spaces.

The presence of doubt does not mean you are falling behind. It often means you are being stretched into something more sophisticated than where you started. The discomfort is the growth.

Doubt gets loudest right before a breakthrough. Keep going.

Affirmation

When Doubt Gets Loud

Doubt is not evidence of my inability — it is evidence that I am
being stretched. I choose to measure my progress honestly, not
through comparison. I have come further than doubt wants me to
remember.

Pause & Consider

When Doubt Gets Loud

• What has doubt been saying to you this week? Write it down — and then write the evidence that contradicts it.
• Who or what are you comparing yourself to? How is that comparison serving you — or not serving you?
• What concrete evidence of your growth can you identify from the past several weeks?
• What would you say to a close friend who was feeling exactly what you are feeling right now?

Standing in the Room Where It Is Real

There are moments in nursing that no amount of preparation fully prepares you for.

The first time you stand in a clinical space with real responsibility. The first time you realize that the person in front of you is not a simulation — they are a human being, trusting you with something precious. The first time the weight of this profession lands not in your mind but in your body.

This happens at every level. The student in their first clinical placement. The new graduate on their first solo shift. The advanced practice nurse in their first independent patient encounter. The nurse leader making their first high-stakes decision. The moment changes shape with each level. The feeling of standing in the room where it is real does not.

You may feel like an imposter in that room. Like everyone around you knows something you do not. Like you are about to be found out. That feeling is one of the most universal experiences in nursing — nearly every nurse you will ever work beside has stood exactly where you are standing and felt exactly what you are feeling.

You belong in that room. You have been prepared for it. Show up attentive, humble, and willing. That is enough for today.

Affirmation

Standing in the Room Where It Is Real

I belong in this space. I arrive prepared, attentive, and willing to learn. I do not need to know everything — I need to be present and accountable. I am becoming the nurse these patients deserve.

Pause & Consider

Standing in the Room Where It Is Real

• What emotions did you experience when the weight of real responsibility landed this week?
• What moment will you carry with you from this week? What did it teach you?
• Where did you surprise yourself with what you already knew or could do?
• What do you want to remember about this week when you are a confident, experienced nurse?

WEEK NINE

Feeling Everything and Still Functioning

Nursing asks something of you that most professions do not: it asks you to feel deeply and still function clearly.

Clinical environments are not calm. They are emotionally layered, fast-moving, and full of human experience at its most raw — fear, pain, grief, relief, loss. And you are in the middle of it, still learning, still becoming, still carrying your own life outside those walls.

Emotional regulation in nursing is not about suppressing what you feel. It is about learning to feel it without letting it drive your decisions. It is about holding what is happening around you without being consumed by it. It is the space between what you witness and what you do next.

This skill develops at every level and through every new clinical experience. It does not arrive fully formed. It builds through the accumulation of difficult moments handled with increasing grace.

What you are experiencing this week — whatever emotional weight you are carrying from a clinical encounter, a patient interaction, a moment that stayed with you after you left — that is not a sign that you are too sensitive for nursing. It is a sign that you are paying attention. The nurses who feel nothing are not the safe ones.

Feel it. Process it. And keep going.

Affirmation

Feeling Everything and Still Functioning

I am allowed to feel deeply and still respond with clarity. My emotional awareness makes me a better nurse. I am learning to hold what I feel without being controlled by it — and that is one of the most important skills I will ever build.

Pause & Consider

Feeling Everything and Still Functioning

• What from this week stayed with you after you left the clinical or learning environment? What did it bring up?
• How did you process that emotional weight? What helped?
• What is the difference between being emotionally present and being emotionally overwhelmed?
• What routines or practices help you reset emotionally so you can keep showing up fully?

WEEK TEN

You Are Not Who You Were

Stop for a moment. Look back.

You are not the same person who began this journey. Whether you started this particular chapter of your nursing path weeks ago or months ago — you have changed. The evidence is in how you think, how you move, how you see.

You notice things now that you would not have noticed before. You ask questions that would not have occurred to you earlier. You carry a kind of awareness that was not there when you began. Clinical language that once felt foreign has become familiar. Skills that once required intense concentration are beginning to feel more natural. Situations that once overwhelmed you are becoming navigable.

This growth does not always feel dramatic. It rarely announces itself. It builds quietly, in the accumulation of days, of practice, of showing up. But it is real. And it deserves to be acknowledged — not just pushed past in the rush toward what comes next.

At every level of nursing, this moment arrives. The moment when you realize you have become something you were not before. Trust it. You have earned it.

You are not who you were. Keep becoming.

Affirmation

You Are Not Who You Were

I have grown in ways I do not always see clearly. The evidence of my becoming is real — in how I think, how I observe, how I show up. I honor the distance I have traveled and I continue forward.

Pause & Consider

You Are Not Who You Were

• Look back at where you began this season. What is genuinely different about you now?
• Where do you notice that you have started thinking or seeing like a nurse — even outside of clinical settings?
• What strength has emerged in you during this season that you did not know you had?
• What do you want to remember about this phase of your journey when you are further along?

WEEK ELEVEN

Professional Presence

Professional presence is not performance. It is not about saying the right things or appearing a certain way for the benefit of an audience. It is about alignment — the quiet integrity of being the same person in the hallway that you are in the patient's room. The same professional when someone is watching that you are when no one is.

At every level of nursing, presence is felt before credentials are verified. Patients sense it. Colleagues recognize it. The nurse who moves through a space with genuine composure, clarity, and care communicates something before a single word is spoken.

You may be navigating environments right now that do not always model the professionalism you are working to develop. Spaces where the standard is not consistently held. Where what is taught in the classroom does not always match what is practiced in the hallway. That dissonance is real — and it is one of the harder parts of nursing formation that no textbook fully addresses.

Here is what I need you to hold onto: your professional standard belongs to you. It is not determined by the environment around you. You are not responsible for how others show up. You are only responsible for how you show up.

Let your presence be the standard you set for yourself — regardless of what surrounds you.

Affirmation

Professional Presence

I carry my integrity into every room I enter. My professional presence belongs to me — it is not dependent on the environment being perfect. I hold my own standard with quiet, consistent excellence.

Pause & Consider

Professional Presence

• What does professional presence look like for you specifically — in your current clinical or learning environment?
• Have you encountered a moment recently where you had to choose between matching the energy around you and holding your own standard? What did you choose?
• What do patients, residents, or colleagues experience when you enter their space? What do you want them to experience?
• What aspect of your professional presence are you most proud of right now?

WEEK TWELVE

Endurance Is a Skill

Nobody talks about this part.

The part where your body is tired in a way that sleep does not fully repair. The part where you have been running at full capacity and the path ahead still stretches further than you can clearly see. The part where you wonder — not about your intelligence or your heart — but about your stamina. Whether you are built to sustain this.

Endurance is not glamorous. It does not look like inspiration. It looks like waking up when every part of you wants to stay. Reviewing when your eyes want to close. Showing up when your body is asking for rest. Choosing — again, and again, and again — to continue.

This is not weakness. This is the work.

Every nurse who has ever stood at a bedside with confidence and competence passed through a season exactly like this one. Not around it. Through it. The endurance you are building in this season is not separate from your clinical formation — it is part of it. The capacity to sustain yourself through difficulty is one of the most important things nursing will ever ask of you.

Keep going. The nurse you are becoming is being forged in exactly this.

Affirmation

Endurance Is a Skill

My tiredness is not weakness — it is evidence of how hard I have
been working. I honor what my body needs and I continue anyway.
Endurance is a skill I am building.
I am stronger than I feel right now.

Pause & Consider

Endurance Is a Skill

• What is your body telling you right now? What does it need that you have not been giving it?
• What is keeping you going on the days when motivation has completely disappeared?
• What is one small, sustainable thing you can do this week to protect your physical and emotional energy?
• When you are a nurse caring for a patient who wants to give up — what will you draw on from this season to help them keep going?

WEEK THIRTEEN

When the Pieces Begin to Connect

Something begins to happen in the middle of every nursing season
that is hard to describe until you experience it.
The pieces start to connect.

What once felt like isolated information begins to speak to itself.
The science connects to the clinical. The communication skills
connect to the assessment findings. The values you studied connect
to what you witnessed in practice. The fragments of knowledge that
once felt separate begin to weave into something coherent.

This is integration. And it is one of the most important
developments in your formation as a nurse — at every level. The
student begins to see how body systems relate to each other. The
experienced nurse begins to see patterns across patient populations.
The advanced practice provider begins to integrate evidence into
complex clinical decisions. The nurse leader begins to see how
individual patient outcomes connect to systemic patterns.

Integration does not require a perfect environment to happen. It
requires your attention, your reflection, and your willingness to
keep making connections between what you are learning and what
you are experiencing.

Trust the process that is happening inside you. The connections are
forming. Even now.

Affirmation

When the Pieces Begin to Connect

I am connecting knowledge to experience in ways I could not
before. My thinking is deepening. I trust the integration taking
place inside me even when I cannot fully see it yet.

Pause & Consider

When the Pieces Begin to Connect

- What concept or skill connected for you this week in a new way? What made that connection happen?
- Where have you surprised yourself with how much you now understand compared to where you started?
- How does your real-world experience help you understand content differently than when you only studied it academically?
- What question are you still sitting with that deserves more of your attention?

WEEK FOURTEEN

When the Weight Gets Personal

Some experiences in nursing stay with you after you leave the building.

A patient whose situation reminded you of someone you love. A resident whose loneliness was palpable. A family in crisis at a bedside. A moment where everything you could do was not enough — and you had to keep going anyway.

Grief in nursing is not talked about enough. Not the clinical kind — the kind where you drive home carrying something you did not carry in with you. Where you find yourself thinking about a person you cared for in the middle of an ordinary moment. Where the sadness does not have a clean name.

That grief is not a problem. It is proof that you showed up fully. It means you were present enough to be affected. And presence — genuine, attentive, human presence — is the foundation of nursing care.

At every level, this weight visits you. It visits the student after their first difficult clinical experience. It visits the seasoned nurse after a patient they knew for years takes a turn. It visits the advanced practice provider after a hard conversation with a family. The weight changes form. It does not go away entirely. Nor should it.

Give yourself permission to feel what you feel. And then, when you are ready, keep going. That is what nurses do.

Affirmation

When the Weight Gets Personal

I am allowed to grieve. My feelings are not weakness — they are evidence of my humanity, which is the foundation of my nursing care. I carry what I have witnessed with tenderness, and I continue forward with purpose.

Pause & Consider

When the Weight Gets Personal

• Has there been a patient, resident, or clinical experience recently that stayed with you after you left? What did it teach you?
• How do you process the emotional weight of nursing? What helps you carry it without being consumed by it?
• What does it mean to you to be fully present with someone who is suffering?
• Who can you talk to when you are carrying something heavy from your clinical experience?

WEEK FIFTEEN

An Honest Inventory

Stop. Just for a moment. Stop.

Before you move forward, you deserve to look back honestly at how far you have come.

Not to judge yourself. Not to calculate what you should have done differently. But to see clearly — with the same honest eyes you bring to a clinical assessment — what is working, what needs adjustment, and what evidence exists that you are growing.

This moment of honest inventory belongs to every nurse at every level. The student at the midpoint of their semester. The new graduate several months into their first position. The advanced practice nurse a year into their new role. The nurse leader mid-way through a major initiative. Every journey has its midpoints. And midpoints deserve honest reflection — not performance, not pretense, but clarity.

What has this season produced in you beyond the measurable outcomes? What habits are serving you? What patterns need to shift? What evidence confirms that you are becoming?

Take an honest inventory. All of it counts.

Affirmation

An Honest Inventory

I look at my progress honestly and without harsh judgment.
Measurable outcomes are one part of my growth — not the whole
story. I acknowledge what I have built, I refine what needs
attention, and I move forward with clarity and intention.

Pause & Consider

An Honest Inventory

• Looking back at the first half of this season, what are you most proud of — not in terms of outcomes, but in terms of who you are becoming?
• What specific habits or practices are serving you well right now? What needs to change?
• What has this season revealed about how you respond to pressure, difficulty, and uncertainty?
• What do you need — professionally, emotionally, physically — to finish this season strong?

WEEK SIXTEEN

Rising Standards

Every nursing journey has a point where the expectations increase.

The content deepens. The clinical reasoning required becomes more sophisticated. The responsibility carried becomes more visible. The margin for error narrows — not to punish you, but because you are developing into someone who can handle less margin.

Rising standards are evidence of growth, not threat. The program or environment that asks more of you does so because you have demonstrated that you are ready for more — even when you do not feel ready.

This happens at every level. The student moves from foundational concepts to complex clinical integration. The nurse moves from following protocols to exercising independent judgment. The advanced practice provider moves from supervised practice to full autonomy. The nurse leader moves from managing tasks to shaping systems.

Each elevation in standard is an invitation — not an accusation. It says: you have grown enough that we are trusting you with more.

You have already met every standard this season has placed in front of you. The evidence is in the fact that you are still here. Let that matter.

Affirmation

Rising Standards

Higher standards are evidence of my growth, not proof of my inadequacy. I have met every challenge placed before me so far. I rise to meet what comes next with the same determination that has carried me to this point.

Pause & Consider

Rising Standards

- Where have the expectations increased recently? How are you adjusting to meet them?
- What preparation habit is serving you best at this higher level of expectation?
- On the days when rising standards feel like too much — what brings you back to center?
- What would it mean for your future patients if you committed fully to these higher standards right now?

Your Voice as a Clinical Tool

Communication is not a soft skill in nursing. It is a clinical safety skill.

The nurse who speaks up clearly — about a concern, an observation, a question, a change in condition — is the nurse who protects patients. The nurse who stays silent, who waits too long, who doubts whether their voice deserves to be heard — that silence has consequences.

At every level of nursing, the voice carries different weight. The student advocates for their own learning. The nurse advocates for their patient's safety. The advanced practice provider advocates in clinical conversations with physicians and specialists. The nurse leader advocates for systems that protect both patients and staff. The form of advocacy changes. The courage required to use your voice does not.

You may have encountered environments where speaking up felt risky. Where you were not sure your question would be welcomed. Where the space did not feel safe for your voice. That experience is real — and it is not your fault.

But here is what I need you to carry forward regardless of what any environment has made you feel: your voice is a clinical instrument. It belongs to your patients. And learning to use it — clearly, respectfully, even when you are afraid — is one of the most important things you will do in nursing.

Affirmation

Your Voice as a Clinical Tool

My voice is a clinical safety tool. I practice using it with clarity and respect. I speak up for my patients, for my learning, and for myself — because silence is never neutral in a clinical environment.

Pause & Consider

Your Voice as a Clinical Tool

• Was there a moment recently when you held back from speaking up? What stopped you? What would you do differently?
• What is the difference between speaking up with composure and speaking up from fear? How do you practice the former?
• How has your communication style changed since you began your nursing journey? What has grown?
• Think of a nurse you have observed who communicates with clarity and confidence. What specifically do they do that you want to develop in yourself?

WEEK EIGHTEEN

Accountability and Ownership

One of the quietest marks of professional maturity is this: the ability to say, clearly and without defensiveness, 'I made an error — and here is what I am doing about it.'

Accountability in nursing is not about punishment. It is about integrity. It is the willingness to look honestly at your actions, acknowledge what went wrong, correct it quickly, and learn thoroughly so it does not happen again.

This is harder than it sounds — especially in environments where admitting uncertainty feels risky. Where asking for help feels like exposing weakness. Where the culture does not always make it safe to say: I am not sure. I need to check. I made a mistake.

But professional ownership is the foundation of safe nursing practice at every level. The student who learns to own their errors in the learning environment becomes the nurse who catches them before they reach patients. The nurse who owns their clinical decisions becomes the leader others can trust. The advanced practice provider who holds themselves accountable becomes the practitioner whose patients are safe.

Build this practice now. In every skill, every assessment, every moment where honesty costs you something. These are the architecture of the nurse you are becoming.

Affirmation

Accountability and Ownership

I take ownership of my growth and my errors with equal honesty.
Accountability is not shame — it is integrity. I correct quickly, learn
thoroughly, and move forward with greater wisdom than I had
before.

Pause & Consider

Accountability and Ownership

• Was there a moment recently where you had to acknowledge an error or uncertainty? How did you handle it?
• What is the difference between accountability and self-punishment? How do you practice one without falling into the other?
• How does professional ownership build trust — with patients, with colleagues, with the people who are counting on you?
• What is the most important thing a difficult moment or mistake has taught you in this season?

WEEK NINETEEN

Learning to See

Something is different now about how you see.
You notice things you would not have noticed before. Details that once passed by unregistered now catch your attention. Patterns that were invisible to you earlier are beginning to emerge. You walk into a space and begin assessing before anyone tells you to.

This is clinical discernment. And it develops at every level of nursing through the accumulation of attention — through every assessment, every observation, every moment of paying careful attention when it would have been easier not to.

The student begins to notice subtle changes in a patient's presentation. The experienced nurse begins to recognize patterns across similar cases. The advanced practice provider begins to synthesize observations into clinical reasoning. The nurse leader begins to see systemic patterns in data that others miss.

You may not fully trust what you are seeing yet. You may notice something and then immediately question yourself — am I right? Should I say something? Trust the observation. Document it. Communicate it. Let the clinical process do the rest.

You are developing the eyes of a nurse. Do not underestimate what that means.

Affirmation

Learning to See

I am learning to see what others might miss. My clinical observations matter and deserve to be spoken. I trust my developing discernment and I act on it with confidence and accountability.

Pause & Consider

Learning to See

• What did you notice this week that you would not have observed earlier in your nursing journey?
• Was there a moment where you observed something and were unsure whether to speak up? What did you do? What would you do now?
• How do you distinguish between a clinical instinct worth reporting and ordinary anxiety?
• What does it mean to you to be the person in the room who truly sees what is happening?

WEEK TWENTY

Carrying Two Things at Once

Right now, many of you are carrying two things simultaneously. You are carrying the demands of this season — the academic, clinical, and professional expectations that keep coming regardless of what else is happening in your life.

And you are carrying something quieter. The emotional residue of this journey. The weight of what you have witnessed. The interactions that stayed with you. The grief, the doubt, the frustration, the moments of genuine connection, the exhaustion that lives underneath everything.

You are carrying both. At the same time. Without being able to put one down in order to manage the other.

That is not ordinary. That is the specific and extraordinary burden of becoming a nurse — at every level, in every season. You do not get to separate the clinical from the human. They are always both present. And learning to hold both — to function clearly while feeling deeply — is one of the most important things nursing will ever ask of you.

You are already doing it. Give yourself credit for that.

Affirmation

Carrying Two Things at Once

I acknowledge the full weight of what I am carrying — clinical,
emotional, personal. I do not minimize it. I honor it.
And I continue forward because I know that what I am building is
worth the weight.

Pause & Consider

Carrying Two Things at Once

• What are you carrying right now that has nothing to do with your clinical or academic performance but everything to do with your formation as a nurse?
• How have you managed carrying multiple demands simultaneously in this season?
• What has this season asked of you that you did not know you were capable of giving?
• What does it mean to you that you are still here, still going, even after everything this season has held?

Professional Identity

At some point, something shifts.

The work begins to feel less like assignments and more like responsibility. You start to recognize the nurse you are becoming—not only through skill, but through character, judgment, and commitment to the people you serve.

This stage is about recognizing that professional identity is not built in a single moment, but through steady growth, reflection, and the courage to keep learning.

Advocacy With Composure

You have been studying advocacy. Now let us talk about what it actually looks like when the environment is difficult.

Advocacy is not always loud. It is not always confrontational. Sometimes it looks like writing a clear, respectful email and pressing send. Sometimes it looks like documenting an interaction carefully — without embellishment, without emotion — so the record is accurate. Sometimes it looks like walking to a trusted person's office and saying quietly: I need to tell you something.

Advocacy at every level of nursing requires the same core skills: clarity, documentation, composure, and the willingness to use the appropriate channels even when it would be easier to stay silent.

The student who learns to advocate for themselves in the learning environment becomes the nurse who advocates for their patients without hesitation. The nurse who learns to raise concerns through proper channels becomes the leader who builds systems that protect everyone. Advocacy, practiced early, becomes instinct.

You have more tools for advocacy than you may realize. And you have been using some of them already — every time you named what you experienced honestly, every time you sought support rather than suffering alone, every time you chose to continue rather than disappear.

Your voice deserves to be used. Use it with composure. Use it with documentation. Use it without apology.

Affirmation

Advocacy With Composure

I advocate for myself and my patients with clarity, documentation,
and composure. My voice is a professional instrument. I use it
strategically, respectfully, and without apology.

Pause & Consider

Advocacy With Composure

• Think of a moment recently where you advocated for yourself or a patient. What did that look like? How did it feel?
• What does composure add to advocacy that emotion alone cannot provide?
• If you needed to raise a concern in your current environment, what would you say and to whom? What documentation would support that conversation?
• How does learning to advocate for yourself now prepare you to advocate for patients who cannot speak for themselves?

WEEK TWENTY-TWO

You Are Not Starting Over

As this season approaches its closing weeks, some of you are beginning to think about what comes next. A new course. A new clinical rotation. A new role. A new level. And with those thoughts can come a feeling that is hard to name — something like anxiety, something like grief, something like beginning again.

I want to say something clearly: you are not starting over. Everything you have built in this season — the clinical judgment, the communication skills, the emotional endurance, the professional identity forming quietly beneath the surface — that travels with you. It is yours. It cannot be taken away by a new classroom, a new floor, a harder course, a more complex patient population.

You will walk into the next season different from how you walked into this one. More grounded. More self-aware. More capable of recognizing what you need and how to get it. The work of this season has prepared you for exactly what is coming next.

At every level of nursing, what you have built accumulates. Nothing is wasted. Every difficult season has deposited something in you that the next season will call upon.

You are not starting over. You are starting from here.

Affirmation

You Are Not Starting Over

I do not start over — I start from here. Everything I have built this season belongs to me and travels with me. I enter what comes next stronger, clearer, and more grounded than I have ever been.

Pause & Consider

You Are Not Starting Over

• What are you carrying forward from this season that you did not
have when you started?
• What concerns you most about the next phase of your journey?
What would help ease that concern?
• What has this season taught you about how you handle new,
difficult, or unfamiliar situations?
• If you could give advice to the version of yourself who began this
season, what would you say?

WEEK TWENTY-THREE

Emotional Maturity

Emotional maturity is not the absence of emotion. It is not the face that never shows strain or the professional who seems untouched by what surrounds them.

Emotional maturity is the space between what happens to you and what you do next. It is the ability to feel what is real — frustration, grief, fear, anger, overwhelm — and still choose how you respond. It develops through exactly the kinds of experiences this season has given you.

You have been in situations where the appropriate emotional response was strong — and you had to manage it anyway. You may have felt dismissed and had to continue professionally. You may have witnessed suffering and had to keep functioning. You may have received feedback that felt unfair and had to receive it without losing your composure. You may have navigated an environment that tested your dignity and had to hold your standard regardless.

That is not suppression. That is regulation. And regulation — knowing how to hold what you feel without being controlled by it — is one of the most critical clinical skills you will ever develop.

You have been developing it all season. In every hard moment. Every time you chose your response over your reaction. Give yourself credit for that.

Affirmation

Emotional Maturity

I feel deeply and respond with intention. My emotional awareness makes me a better nurse. I have learned to hold what I feel without being controlled by it — and that is a skill I will carry for the rest of my career.

Pause & Consider

Emotional Maturity

• What situation in this season required the most emotional regulation from you? How did you manage it?
• What is the difference between suppressing your emotions and regulating them? Which are you practicing?
• How has your emotional response to difficult situations changed since you began your nursing journey?
• When a patient or family member triggers a strong emotional response in you, what will you draw on from this season?

WEEK TWENTY-FOUR

Identity Stabilizing

You are no longer who you were when you began.

Somewhere in the middle of all the studying and clinical experiences and evaluations and emotional weight of this season, a professional identity has been forming. Quietly. Without announcement. Shaped by every decision you made when no one was watching. Every moment you chose integrity over convenience. Every time you showed up when you could have found a reason not to.

That identity — the nurse you are becoming — is yours. It was not given to you by a grade or an evaluation or a title. It was built by you, through the accumulation of this season.

It may still feel uncertain. Professional identity stabilizes over time, not all at once. But it is there. You can sense it in how you carry yourself in clinical spaces. In how you think about patients. In how you understand your own strengths and limitations. In the values that are becoming non-negotiable for you.

At every level of nursing, this stabilizing happens. The student begins to feel like a nurse. The nurse begins to feel like a professional. The advanced practice provider begins to feel like a clinician. The leader begins to feel like a steward of the profession.

You are becoming. And what you are becoming is real.

Affirmation

Identity Stabilizing

My professional identity is forming — quietly, patiently, through
every choice I have made this season.
I do not need it to be fully formed to trust its direction.
I am becoming a nurse.
And that becoming is already visible.

Pause & Consider

Identity Stabilizing

• How would you describe the nurse you are becoming? Not your skills — your character. What words come to mind?
• What moment this season most clearly showed you who you are as a developing nursing professional?
• How does your professional identity feel different now than it did when you began?
• What value or principle is at the core of the nurse you are becoming? Where did it come from?

The Finish Line Is Not the End

The end of this season is close enough now that you can feel it.

And with that feeling comes something complicated. Relief. Exhaustion. A pride that has not fully settled yet. And for some of you — fear. Fear about whether you performed well enough. Fear about what comes next. For some, the possibility that this season may not end the way you hoped.

I want to speak directly to that fear.

If you are in a place where you are uncertain about outcomes — please know this: this is not the end of your story. It is a moment of recalibration. Some of the most extraordinary nurses in practice today did not move through their journey in a straight line. They repeated courses. They changed directions. They took longer than expected. And they became extraordinary because of — not in spite of — the detours.

The finish line of this season is not the final measure of your worth as a nurse. It is one marker on a much longer path. What matters most is not how this season ends — it is what you learned, how you grew, and whether you are still committed to continuing.

The path continues. Keep walking.

Affirmation

The Finish Line Is Not the End

Whether this season ends as I hoped or asks me to recalibrate, I am still becoming. My path does not have to be straight to be real. I move forward from wherever I land with honesty, dignity, and determination.

Pause & Consider

The Finish Line Is Not the End

• Where do you stand right now in this season? What specific action can you take today to strengthen your position before it ends?
• If you are facing an unexpected outcome, who can you speak to about your options? Have you had that conversation yet?
• What do you know about yourself as a learner now that you did not know when you began?
• Regardless of outcomes, what has this season built in you that no evaluation can measure?

When the Outcome Was Not What You Worked For

Some experiences in nursing cannot be fully prepared for. Even when you have studied every possibility, practiced every skill, and given everything you have — sometimes the outcome is not what you worked for.

A patient declines despite excellent care. A clinical decision does not produce the expected result. A procedure does not go as planned. A conversation with a family does not bring the comfort you intended. The outcome falls short of what the effort deserved.

This happens at every level of nursing. And it is one of the hardest things the profession asks of you: to care fully, to give everything, and to accept that not every outcome is within your control.

The question 'did I do everything I could?' is an important one. Ask it. Reflect on it honestly. Let it sharpen your practice. But when the honest answer is 'yes' — let yourself receive that. Guilt that is not grounded in error is not accountability. It is grief. And grief deserves to be treated gently.

You are learning one of the most profound lessons nursing teaches: how to care without guarantees. How to give fully knowing that giving fully is sometimes not enough. And how to keep showing up anyway — because the next patient needs the nurse you are still becoming.

Affirmation

When the Outcome Was Not What You Worked For

I reflect honestly on difficult outcomes without carrying blame that is not mine to hold. I learn from what I can control and release what I cannot.
Caring fully — even when the outcome is hard — is the highest expression of nursing.

Pause & Consider

*When the Outcome Was Not What
You Worked For*

• Has there been an experience recently where the outcome was not what you hoped, despite your best effort? How did you process it?
• What is the difference between learning from a difficult outcome and punishing yourself for it?
• How do you hold grief and professionalism simultaneously? What does that look like for you?
• Who have you talked to about the emotionally difficult parts of your clinical experience? Is there someone you trust with that weight?

WEEK TWENTY-SEVEN

Looking Ahead With Composure

It is natural to look ahead. To think about what comes next. To begin mentally preparing for the next season, the next level, the next chapter.

But before you move forward, I want to invite you to stay here for just a moment longer. Because here — in these final weeks of this particular season — there is still something worth witnessing.

You made it through something that mattered. Not just academically or professionally. Personally. You showed up for patients while carrying your own weight. You continued learning in environments that were not always easy. You found people to trust and leaned on them carefully. You grew braver as the season got harder. You held your standard when holding it cost you something.

That is the story of this season. And it deserves to be acknowledged — fully, honestly, with the same presence you have brought to every difficult moment — before you carry it forward.

Look ahead with composure. Not with the anxious energy of someone running away from where they have been. But with the grounded confidence of someone who knows what they have survived and what they have built.

You are ready for what comes next. Because you have already proven you can do hard things.

Affirmation

Looking Ahead With Composure

I honor where I am before I move forward. I look ahead not with
anxiety but with the grounded confidence of someone who has
already proven they can do hard things.
I am ready for what comes next.

Pause & Consider

Looking Ahead With Composure

• What are you most looking forward to about the next phase of your nursing journey?
• What concern about what comes next feels biggest right now? What information or support would help?
• How do you want to carry yourself into the next season — what do you want to bring, and what do you want to leave behind?
• What has this season taught you about who you can go to when you need support?

The Final Stretch

You are in the final stretch.

Everything that remains requires the specific kind of energy that only comes from knowing the end is near and choosing to finish with the same integrity you started with. Not the explosive energy of a new beginning. The steady, deliberate energy of someone who has come too far to give anything less than their best.

Some of your bodies are speaking to you differently now. The sustained effort of this season has a physical signature — a kind of tiredness that lives deeper than sleep can reach. Some of you have gotten sick. Some of you are running on determination and the quiet knowledge that you are almost there.

Honor your body. And keep going.

Do not cut corners in these final days. Do not give anything less than your full presence to the patients, residents, and people in your care. The person you are serving in the final week of this season deserves the same fully present nurse as the one in your first week.

Finish the way you started. With courage, with care, and with everything you have.

Affirmation

The Final Stretch

I finish what I start — with the same integrity and care I brought on
the first day.
Those I serve in these final days deserve my full presence.
I give it gladly because it is who I am becoming.

Pause & Consider

The Final Stretch

- What does your body need right now to get through the final stretch? What can you give it, even imperfectly?
- What is the most important thing you need to do this week to finish well?
- How do you want to show up in your final clinical or professional days of this season?
- What will it mean to you to complete this season? Take a moment to imagine it fully.

What You Know Now

There are things you know now that you could not have known at the beginning of this season.

You know what it feels like to carry real responsibility in your body. You know what clinical or professional fatigue feels like. You know what it means to care for someone who is suffering and to keep going anyway. You know what it feels like to question yourself — and to slowly, carefully, begin to trust yourself.

You know what kind of environment helps you grow. You know what support looks like when it is real. You know the difference between a space that builds you and one that asks you to protect yourself. You know how to ask for help — and you know that asking is strength, not weakness.

This self-knowledge is not a small thing. It will inform every clinical decision, every professional relationship, every leadership moment that comes next. The nurse who knows themselves is the nurse whose patients are safe — because self-knowledge means knowing your strengths, knowing your limits, and acting accordingly.

Carry this self-knowledge forward. It is one of the most valuable things this season has given you.

Affirmation

What You Know Now

What I have learned this season goes far beyond clinical content. I have learned about myself — how I grow, what I need, and what I am capable of. I carry that self-knowledge forward as one of the most valuable tools I own.

Pause & Consider

What You Know Now

• What do you know about yourself as a nursing professional that you could not have known before this season?
• What kind of environment helps you grow most? How will you seek that out going forward?
• What do you want to remember about being a learner in this season — when you are in a position to support others?
• How has this season changed what you believe about the kind of nurse you are capable of becoming?

WEEK THIRTY

Grace Under Pressure

Nursing will ask you to operate under pressure for the rest of your career. That is not a warning. It is simply the nature of the work.

Clinical environments are fast, unpredictable, and emotionally layered. They ask you to think clearly when clarity is hard. To communicate precisely when the stakes are high. To remain composed when everything around you is urgent. To hold your standard when the environment is not holding its own.

Grace under pressure is not something you are born with. It is something you build — through exactly the kinds of experiences this season has given you.

You have operated under pressure this season. In conditions that were sometimes harder than they needed to be. In moments where the external environment was not supporting you the way it should have. And you held your standard anyway. You showed up with integrity. You continued becoming.

That is grace under pressure. And the nurses who develop it — who learn early what it means to maintain their standard regardless of what surrounds them — become the steady, trusted presence that patients and teams depend on for an entire career.

You are building that presence. Right now. In these hardest weeks.

Affirmation

Grace Under Pressure

I have demonstrated grace under pressure this season. My standard
does not depend on the environment meeting mine. I carry my
integrity with me into every space — and that is the foundation of
the nurse I am becoming.

Pause & Consider

Grace Under Pressure

• Where have you demonstrated grace under pressure this season
— in ways you may not have fully credited yourself for?
• What has this season taught you about maintaining your standard
even when the environment falls short?
• How do you want to be known by your patients as a nurse? What
character traits define that vision?
• What is the most important thing this season has built in you that
will make you a better nurse than you would have been without it?

WEEK THIRTY-ONE

The Nurses Who Come After You

There are nursing students beginning their journey right now who do not know you exist.

Who will walk into a learning environment for the first time carrying the same hope, the same anxiety, the same questions you carried when you began. Who will face some of the same challenges you have faced. Who will wonder, in their hardest weeks, whether they belong in this profession.

Because of what you have been through this season — because of what you endured, what you learned, what you survived with your integrity intact — they will have something you may not have had.

They will have nurses like you.

The nurses who remember what it felt like to be a student in a difficult environment are the nurses who make sure their students never feel alone in it. The nurses who learned to advocate for themselves become the nurses who teach others to do the same. The nurses who survived hard seasons with grace become the ones who create better environments for the generations that follow.

Your story is still being written. But already, the way you are becoming is doing something good in the world — even if you cannot see it yet.

Affirmation

The Nurses Who Come After You

My journey through this season matters beyond my own experience. The way I am becoming will extend to nurses and students I have not yet met.
My becoming is already making a difference.

Pause & Consider

The Nurses Who Come After You

• What would you want the next generation of nursing students to know about what this season was like — and what got you through it?
• What advice would you give to someone just beginning the season you are completing?
• What does it mean to you that your experience — including the hard parts — has the potential to help someone else?
• How do you want to contribute to the culture of nursing as a colleague, a mentor, and a presence in the profession?

WEEK THIRTY-TWO

Professional Integration

The student and the nurse are becoming the same person.

That is one of the most remarkable things that happens as a nursing season comes to a close — this quiet merging of who you have been in the learning environment and who you are becoming in practice. The professional identity that felt separate from your 'real self' at the beginning has slowly integrated. You think like a nurse now. You carry a clinical awareness that was not there before. You process the world differently.

This integration does not happen all at once. But you can feel it. The way you move in clinical spaces with more confidence than anxiety. The way clinical language has become natural. The way you look at a person and begin to see them clinically before anyone tells you to.

You are not performing nursing anymore. You are beginning to simply be a nurse.

This is true at every level. The student becomes a nurse. The nurse becomes a professional. The advanced practice provider becomes a clinician. The nurse leader becomes a steward. At each level, a new integration occurs — a deeper merging of self and role.

The nurse you are becoming is already visible. Can you see yourself?

Affirmation

Professional Integration

The nurse I am becoming is already visible. My professional identity
and my personal identity are integrating into something whole. I
am not performing nursing — I am beginning to simply be a nurse.

Pause & Consider

Professional Integration

• Where do you notice that you have started thinking or seeing like a nurse — even outside of clinical settings?
• What skill or habit has become most natural to you that felt completely foreign when you began?
• How would the people who have worked with you this season describe your growth?
• What does the nurse you are becoming look like? Describe this nurse in as much detail as you can.

WEEK THIRTY-THREE

What Was Forging All Along

Looking back now — from where you stand in these final days — can you see it?

The season that asked so much of you. The clinical experiences that stayed with you. The patients and residents whose faces you will carry. The moments of doubt and the moments of certainty. The weeks when you were afraid and the weeks when you were steady. The times you found your voice and the times you held it strategically, waiting for the right moment.

All of it — every single week — was forging something.

Not breaking you. Forging you. The way intense heat and sustained pressure forge something raw into something refined, purposeful, and strong. You are not the same person who began this season. The work of these weeks has changed the shape of you.

And what was being forged all along was not just a nursing student, or a nurse, or a practitioner, or a leader. It was a person of integrity. A person who knows what it means to show up when it is hard. A person who has already proven that they can hold the weight of this profession with grace.

That person is you. They were always in you. This season simply revealed you more clearly.

Affirmation

What Was Forging All Along

This season was not just something I survived — it was something
that forged me. Every difficult week, every hard moment, every time
I chose to continue was shaping the nurse I was always becoming.
I am grateful for what the fire made.

Pause & Consider

What Was Forging All Along

• What has this season forged in you that you could not have developed any other way?
• What are you most grateful for from this season — including the parts that were hard?
• Who supported you through this season in ways you have not yet fully acknowledged? How can you honor that?
• What do you want to say to yourself — honestly, warmly — about what you accomplished this season?

WEEK THIRTY-FOUR

The Nurse You Are Becoming

You made it.

However this season ends — with honors or with relief, with a celebration or a quiet exhale, with next steps clearly mapped or still being discerned — you made it through something real. Something that asked everything of you. Something that will matter for the rest of your career.

As you close this reflection companion — or set it down for now, knowing you may return to it at the start of the next season — I want to leave you with something that is not advice and not instruction. Simply truth.

The nursing profession needs you. Not a perfect version of you. Not a version of you that never doubted, never struggled, never sat in your car after a hard day and felt the weight of all of it. You. The real you. The one who showed up anyway.

The patients who will be in your care — they do not need a nurse who has never been afraid. They need a nurse who knows what fear feels like and can hold space for theirs. They do not need a nurse who has never grieved. They need a nurse who has carried loss and kept caring. They need a nurse who has learned to advocate when advocacy is hard. They need a nurse who knows their voice is a clinical tool.

They need you.

The nurse you are becoming — you were here in the very first week,
even when you could not see yourself clearly. You have been
growing steadily through every week of this experience, through
every clinical experience, through every hard moment and quiet
triumph and ordinary day where nothing dramatic happened but
formation continued anyway. You belong in this profession. You
always did.

Go gracefully. Go grounded. You are the nurse you are becoming.

Affirmation

The Nurse You Are Becoming

I have done more than complete a season. I have been formed. I
carry forward everything this journey has built — the knowledge,
the compassion, the courage, the voice, and the unshakeable belief
that I belong in this profession.
The nurse I am becoming is already within me. Always has been.

Pause & Consider

The Nurse You Are Becoming

- What is the most important thing this entire experience has taught you about the nurse you are becoming?
- What do you want to carry with you from this season into every clinical environment you will enter for the rest of your career?
- What do you want to release — what weight, what doubt, what fear — that you no longer need to carry?
- What would you say to the version of yourself who opened this guided reflection companion for the very first time?

CLOSING REFLECTION

Throughout this journey, you have studied skills, practiced discipline, and faced moments that required courage. Some days may have felt uncertain, and other days may have reminded you exactly why you chose this path.

Some of you navigated more than coursework this semester. Some of you carried things that had nothing to do with nursing school and everything to do with becoming a nurse — weight that never appeared on a syllabus but showed up in every clinical day, every exam week, every moment you had to keep going when everything in you wanted to stop. That weight was real. And you carried it with more grace than you may realize.

Becoming a nurse is not formed in a single moment. It develops gradually — through reflection, responsibility, and the willingness to grow through each experience placed before you. The work you have done throughout these pages represents more than assignments completed or weeks finished. It reflects the development of judgment, compassion, and integrity that will shape the way you care for others.

As you move forward in your education and into the profession, remember that the qualities that sustain great nurses are not only knowledge and skill — but also humility, steadiness, and the commitment to continue learning and continue becoming.

The journey you began in these pages is still unfolding. Continue showing up with care, professionalism, and courage for the work ahead.

A Final Word

My first cohort of nursing students does not know they made this experience possible. They showed up determined, navigated more than any student should have to navigate, grew braver as the season got harder, and came through the other side as nurses in the making.

This guided reflection companion exists because of them. Every page was written with their faces in my mind — and with the faces of every nurse who will come after them, at every level, in every season, carrying the same hope and the same extraordinary capacity to become.

You are one of those nurses.

I see you. I have always seen you. And I wrote every word of this for you.

— Nancy S. Ferrell Jones, DNP, RN

FINAL PAUSE

Recognizing Who You Are Now

You have reached the end of this chapter. Not the end of learning — but the end of becoming unfamiliar with yourself.

What once felt overwhelming has become navigable. What once required constant effort now carries rhythm. You no longer question whether you belong here — you move as someone who knows.

Along the way, you learned how to work through fatigue. How to hold responsibility without losing yourself. How to remain steady in environments that were not always steady in return. How to show up — again and again — even when showing up cost you something.

That is not small. That is the foundation of a nurse.

Before you move into the pages that follow — which will reflect back to you what was quietly forming all along — take a moment here. Breathe. Look back honestly at the distance you have traveled since Week One. Not to judge it. Not to grade it. Simply to see it.

You have become someone new. And what was building that becoming deserves to be witnessed before you carry it forward.

FINAL REFLECTION

What I Take With Me

What moments from this journey changed how I see myself as a nurse—and as a person?

What challenges strengthened me in ways I did not expect?

Where did I learn to trust my judgment, even when reassurance was limited?

What values now guide how I show up in clinical spaces, classrooms, and conversations?

What parts of myself do I commit to protecting as I move forward?

FINAL AFFIRMATION

You Are Ready to Continue

You are not leaving this experience the same way you entered it.

You carry discernment now.
You carry steadiness.
You carry the ability to move forward without constant confirmation.

You learned how to listen—to patients, to environments, and to yourself.

You learned when to ask, when to pause, and when to act.

You are allowed to take pride in this work.
You are allowed to rest after effort.
You are allowed to trust what you know.

What comes next will ask new things of you—
but it will not ask you to disappear.

Go forward prepared.
Go forward capable.
Go forward whole.

HOW YOU SHOWED UP

You showed up with integrity — even when guidance was unclear. You chose to do what was right, not what was easiest.

You showed up with questions, not silence. Learning does not require shrinking.

You showed up with compassion — including for yourself. You understood that care begins inward before it extends outward.

You showed up with discernment. You learned the difference between authority and wisdom.

You showed up with steadiness. Not because the path was gentle — but because you learned how to remain whole while walking it.

You showed up. Again and again. Even when it cost you something.

That is who you are.

AND NOW, YOU CONTINUE

You have what you need.

Not because the path ahead will be easy,
but because you have learned how to carry yourself through difficulty
with clarity and care.

This experience was never meant to hold you here.
It was meant to remind you of who you are when you move forward.

Take what serves you.
Return when you need to remember.
Leave the rest behind.

Go gently.
Go grounded.
Keep becoming.

RELEASE

You have done more than complete a semester. You have grown. You have learned how to stand when things felt uncertain. You have learned how to listen to yourself. You have learned that your voice is steady — even when your hands tremble.

You do not leave this season the same way you entered it.

Whether you are stepping forward into the next semester, or stepping back to gather your strength before returning — you do not leave unchanged. You leave wiser. More self-aware. More certain of what you are made of than you were before.

You leave stronger. Clearer. More aware of who you are becoming.

Carry what served you. Release what did not. Walk forward without apology.

The nurse you are becoming is already within you.
Always was.

CARRY THIS WITH YOU

The content you learned this semester will evolve. Protocols will change. Clinical guidelines will be updated. The science of nursing will continue to advance. What you know today will grow into something more sophisticated over time.

But what you built in these pages — the self-awareness, the professional identity, the courage to ask questions and advocate for yourself and your patients — that does not expire. It does not become outdated. It travels with you into every clinical environment you will ever enter.

Whether you are a CNA still working toward nursing school, a first-semester student beginning again next term, or a nurse standing at a bedside years from now — these values belong to you. Carry them with care.

You showed up for this journey. You gave it your honesty. You gave it your effort. And in return, it gave you something no exam can measure — a clearer sense of the nurse you are becoming.

That nurse is already within you.

Professional Guidance

The journey through nursing school is not meant to be walked alone.

The following pages offer guidance, encouragement, and practical direction for moments when you may need clarity, reassurance, or support.

Whether you are navigating a difficult situation, seeking professional guidance, or simply pausing to reflect, remember that asking for help and seeking wisdom are part of becoming a strong and ethical nurse.

If You Ever Need a Safe Next Step

In academic and clinical environments, there may be moments when something does not feel right — whether it is a concern about professionalism, communication, how students are being treated, or the safety of the learning environment itself.

When that happens, it is important to remember: you are not expected to handle it alone. And you do not have to.

Most nursing programs — at every level, whether community college, university, or graduate program — have designated leaders whose responsibility is to receive student concerns with care, professionalism, and discretion. Seeking guidance is not a sign of weakness. It is an act of professional advocacy. For yourself. And for every student who comes after you.

Sometimes the first step is simply beginning the conversation. You do not need the perfect words. You do not need to explain why it took time to speak up. You do not need permission to seek guidance.

A short, respectful message marked confidential is enough to begin. Here is an example:

> Dear [Program Director / Department Chair],
>
> I would appreciate the opportunity to speak privately regarding a concern within the program. When you have time available, I would be grateful for a confidential conversation.
>
> Thank you for your guidance.

In most nursing programs, appropriate points of contact include:

- Nursing Program Director
- Department Chair or Dean of Nursing (if further review is needed)
- Student Services or Academic Advising (for academic concerns)

Nursing is a profession built on advocacy — first for patients, and also for one another. Learning when and how to seek support is one of the quiet ways nurses protect the integrity of the profession and the dignity of those within it.

You deserve a learning environment that reflects the standards of the profession you are entering. And if that environment falls short — you have every right, and every responsibility, to say so through the appropriate channels.

Your voice matters here too.

THE STANDARD OF PROFESSIONAL NURSING

Professional standards guide how nurses care for patients — and how they treat one another. Both matter. Both are part of what it means to be a nurse.

Nursing education is rigorous and demanding. Within that rigor, a culture has developed over generations that you may already have encountered. It is sometimes described with the phrase: nurses eat their young.

This phrase describes a pattern of professional incivility — experienced nurses treating those newer to the profession in ways that diminish rather than develop them. It can begin quietly. Not always in obvious ways. Sometimes it is only recognized later — when the emotional weight of an interaction lingers longer than the lesson itself.

You do not have to accept this as simply 'how nursing is.' It is not how nursing has to be. And it is not the standard the profession holds for itself.

If you encounter conduct that does not align with professional standards, refer to the guidance on the previous page for your next steps.

You deserve a learning environment that prepares you to be the nurse the profession needs.

NOTE FOR FACULTY

This guided companion was designed as a reflection framework for nursing students as they move through the academic and emotional demands of their program. The weekly reflections align with the rhythm of a semester — from early adjustment and foundational discipline to professional awareness, clinical discernment, and identity formation.

Faculty may incorporate the framework in several ways. Some programs invite students to complete one reflection each week, while others integrate selected weeks into seminar discussions, clinical preparation, or leadership courses. The guide may also be used in nursing residency programs, student orientation, or academic advising conversations.

The goal is not to add workload but to create structured space for reflection and professional growth. When students are given consistent space to reflect on their development, they build not only clinical competence but the confidence to participate fully — and to advocate effectively — within their learning environment.
Over time, these reflections help students recognize the formation already taking place within them. They begin to see their growth clearly, name their strengths accurately, and move through the demands of nursing education with greater anchorage and self-awareness.

This companion is designed to be used at any level — community college, university, or graduate nursing programs. It speaks to the nursing student, the aspiring nurse, and the practicing nurse who is still becoming.

Thank you for the work you do in shaping the next generation of nurses. Your presence in the classroom matters more than any textbook can capture.

ABOUT THE AUTHOR

Dr. Nancy S. Ferrell Jones was shaped long before she ever set foot in a nursing program.

She grew up near Fort Campbell, Kentucky — a military community rooted in service, sacrifice, and doing right by others. Her great-grandfather served in World War II. Her grandfather and father carried that legacy of service forward. And her grandparents, who helped raise her, built a home filled with large family gatherings, dancing, joy, good cooking, and hard work.

Life was taught in that home. Not through lectures — through living. Through watching. Through the bold, consistent example of people who knew how to celebrate together and how to carry themselves with dignity when the world got hard.

Her mother — a woman of extraordinary warmth, quiet endurance, and hard-won resilience — taught her what survival looks like from the inside. That lesson became the foundation of how she shows up for every student, every patient, and every nurse still becoming.

That foundation never left her.

Dr. Ferrell Jones began her healthcare journey not in a classroom — but on the floor, as a Certified Nurse Aide on a skilled nursing unit. For nearly a decade, she worked bedside while simultaneously pursuing her undergraduate degrees — holding onto a vision of leadership while doing the work most people overlook.

She earned her Bachelor of Arts in Psychology with a concentration in Natural Science from the University of Louisville and her Bachelor of Science in Nursing from Spalding University. She went on to complete her Doctor of Nursing Practice in Executive Leadership at Capella University, with her practicum placement at Vanderbilt University Medical Center.

Today, she brings more than 25 years of experience spanning clinical care, population health, healthcare consulting, and nursing education. She is the Founder and CEO of beePrestige Healthcare Consulting, where she supports healthcare professionals and organizations in strengthening leadership capacity, clinical integrity, and human-centered systems of care. She is among a small and growing number of Black nurses who hold a Doctor of Nursing Practice degree with a concentration in executive leadership — a distinction that shapes both her perspective and her mission.

She is a member of the American Nurses Association, Sigma Theta Tau International Honor Society of Nursing, American Legion Auxiliary, National League of Nursing, and Alpha Kappa Alpha Sorority, Incorporated. In 2024, she was awarded Spalding University's Caritas Gold Medal — the institution's highest alumni honor — in recognition of her life of innovative leadership and charitable service.

She is also a Nashville Voice, recognized by the Nashville Public Library for her commitment to her community.

The Nurse I Am Becoming is her first book. It was not written from theory. It was written from witness — from standing beside nursing students in their most vulnerable and most courageous moments, and understanding, from personal experience, what it means to keep becoming in a profession that asks everything of you.

She writes for every nursing student who has ever felt the weight of
this journey — and needed someone to help them carry it, week by
week. For those navigating spaces that were not always built to hold
them. And for those who believe — as her family taught her long ago
around tables full of food, laughter, and life — that how we show up for
one another matters more than almost anything else.

> **"Our journey to success is not our own, but by
> the service and sacrifices of those
> bestowed upon us; therefore, it is our duty
> to pay it forward with grace and gratitude."**
> — Dr. Nancy Shataun Ferrell Jones

Connect with Dr. Jones:

beePrestige Healthcare Consulting | www.beeprestigeconsulting.com